HAVE YOU EVER WONDERED WHY OR HOW ESSENTIAL OILS ARE SO EFFECTIVE?

Have you ever wondered why or how Essential Oils are so effective? Is it simply the aroma or is there something more? This book explains how the energetic properties that exist in Essential Oils - and everything else - is the reason why they are so successful in providing relaxation and purification. Everything in the universe possesses an energetic value, including yourself. And this energy effects us, and through the method I am about to present you, you will learn how to balance your energy using Essential Oils and Aromatherapy in a calculated and effective way.

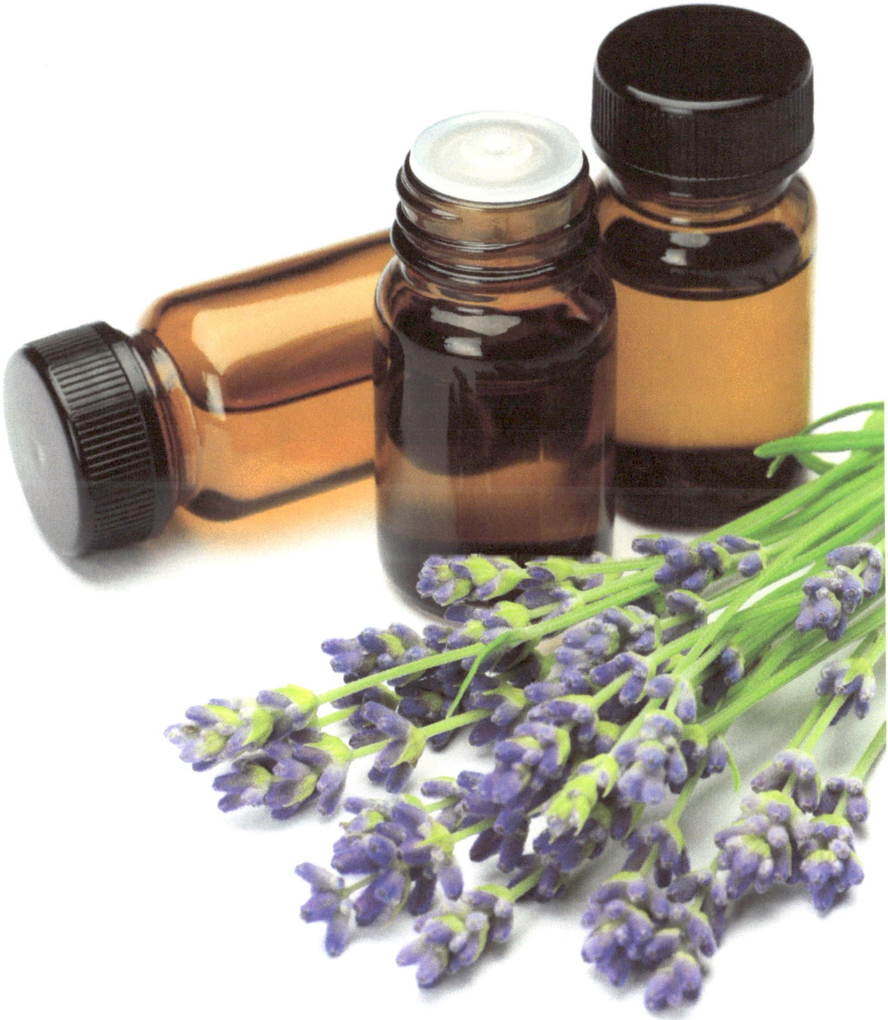

1. THE ENERGY SPECTRUM EXPLAINED

Upon each and every interaction you've experienced in your life, both positive and negative feedback has exchanged between you and the other party. How much affect this has upon either of you, depends on a variety of factors. Think about your life - from birth until this moment — you can most likely pinpoint some influence that a few people have directly had upon you and possibly the influence that you have directed toward them, family, friends, significant others, or even complete strangers. We have all had ups and downs, we have all had both positive and negative influences, we have all had both arguments and harmonies with many people. We all have entered a room and felt good or bad vibrations. However there are many other positive and negative influences that many times we don't recognize so obviously. Subtle exchanges of this energy can have a major affect as well, whether we notice them or not. We each take in both the positive and negative which directly influences who we are and who we will become.

Everything in this universe accumulates and dissipates one thing in common; energy. Essential Oils are no different and they are known through clinical research that they give off the highest frequency of any natural substance. This energy value can be measured very accurately. In fact, when you map out the numeric values of Essential Oils you can find a very unique and interesting pattern — a pattern that could not possibly be by chance — that directly links them together, links them to nature and links them to the human race. If you take all 35 Essential Oils referenced in this booklet, their energy adds up exactly to 0. This has similarities with all

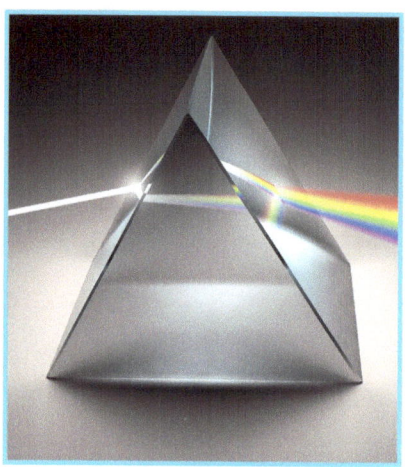

LIGHT REFRACTS THROUGH A PRISM JUST AS ENERGY REFRACTS THROUGH OURSELVES.

of life here on earth and in the heavens; the amount of positive   energy in the universe is exactly the same as the amount of negative energy, giving us a completely balanced zero-energy universe. This can be translated as well with magnetism. The positive and negative charges in magnetism cancel each other out resulting in 0, but it doesn't stop there.

Each human being is like a magnet, with positive and negative charges, either repelling or attracting others' positive and negative charges dependent upon how these ionized electrons interlock together and whether their charges are coequally proportionate. These electrons are affected by natural components - and in particular, the use of natural oils - from the environment that surrounds us. This booklet intends to explain how you can learn the discipline of regulating your energy by use of essential oils as well as interlocking within the energy of others to create a harmony between your entities. Through the power of the relationship between the natural and spiritual worlds, interpersonal equilibrium can be achieved.

Essential Oils carry positive and negative charges, like all things in nature, but through their unique essence, they are the most beneficial and effective external tools in achieving interpersonal equilibrium, when used along with introspection, spiritual guidance, and communication with those who you are teaming with to achieve what I call **0 BALANCE.**

ACHIEVING 0 BALANCE MEANS TO GAIN STABILITY IN ALL ASPECTS, SPIRITUALLY, MENTALLY AND PHYSICALLY

These positive and negative charges have been understood for millennia. In ancient China these were the basis of the Yin and Yang, which was knowledge learned directly from ancient Biblical text. Ancient adepts constructed a system of opposites within opposites that was broken into the 64 trigrams of the I Ching. The 64 trigrams are the same base code as our own computer binary, through which we create virtual worlds with 0's and 1's. We are tapping into this same alchemical process through the olfactory nerves with aromatherapy science. This philosophy has been utilized in a form that is popularly known as Feng Shui. But little has been known of the connection between this union of ancient and modern worlds and the value of the energy-frequency charges of these positive and negative magnetic frequencies, until now, and has proven again that Essential Oils are a link between ancient knowledge, modern knowledge, and the spiritual and physical worlds.

Certain essential oils charge our electrons and ions in various ways, and each of us as individuals need different recipes. One combination of essential oils that may work for you may not work for your sibling, for example. The dependence is not only based on our biology, but our life experience, for we each have been molded and changed independently, based on the positive and negative influences we have endured. Realizing what our chemistry requires to fulfill the equilibrium for which we strive, is realized through self-actualization. This can be achieved through meditation, prayer, and introspection. This book however, intends to give you a guide so that you can rate your energy on a scale so that you have a starting point to re-ionize yourself to intake and give off the correct ratio of positive magnetism to the steady output of negative magnetism.

WE DO NOT PROCURE THE LIGHT OR MAGNETISM, WE ARE THE LIGHT AND MAGNETISM.

EVERYTHING IN THE CREATED UNIVERSE CONSISTS OF ENERGY, INCLUDING US. WE ARE PART OF THIS MAGNIFICENT EXISTENCE, NOT A PASSENGER INSIDE.

ESSENTIAL OILS CAN BIND US TO THIS GREAT MAGNETISM AND ENERGY THAT WE WEILD INSIDE OURSELVES.

WE MUST STRIVE TO ATTAIN BALANCE SO THAT WE CAN MANUEVER WITHIN THIS GREAT EXISTENCE.

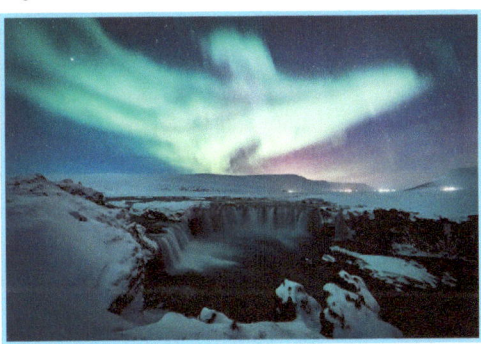

2. MANY PEOPLE MAY ASK, ISN'T ALL NEGATIVE ENERGY HARMFUL?

The answer may surprise you. These terms mean different things in different context. Negative energy as in; someone with a bad attitude or who gives off negative vibrations is not the same as negative magnetism. I implore you to not make the mistake of thinking negative magnetism or the way the term "negative energy" is used in this booklet are harmful vibrations. A magnet cannot exist without both it's positive and negative charge. The negative, is as important as the positive in achieving harmony within oneself, your environment and the universe. Just like your lungs intake beneficial oxygen, and output carbon dioxide, to which the plants use the carbon dioxide to replenish themselves, and thereby are able to create oxygen. It is a cyclic, symbiotic relationship, and thus this symbiosis is recommended for all relationships, not only human to human, but human to plant, human to spirit, spirit to human, and plant to human.

Negative energy is simply the layman explanation of a negative charge or ions, and exists as a counterbalance with positive ions, to create the energy that exists within all life on this planet and beyond, that sit in sliding positions upon an energy scale.

Where we personally fit within this energetic universe can be realized with a simple process of meditation with the graphic in the next chapter. I call this the energy scale, or Energy Spectrum.

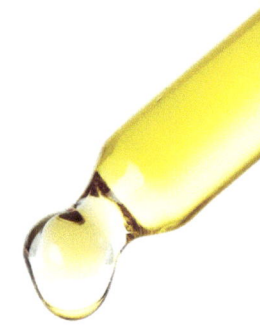

Many researchers in the past, like the late Bruce Tainio. have mapped out biofrequencies to determine the the relationship between frequency and disease, they also measured the frequency of Essential Oils to find a connection. This study parallels those outdated ones, but also has gone beyond them in its findings. In the old studies, they were only able to measure in megahertz, whereas the Energy Spectrum accounts for megahertz, but also incorporates the Planck's Law as well as the Planck-Einstein Energy-Frequency Relation. By introducing these two well known constants of quantum studies, The Energy Spectrum has given accurate results to account for energy values, and not just megahertz.

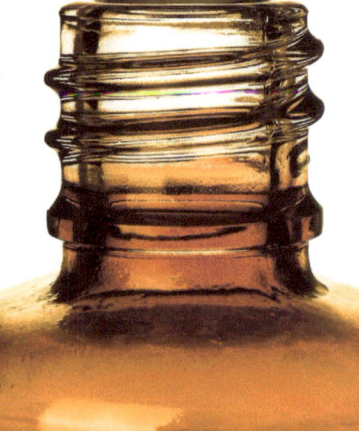

I intend to explain these findings here, however I understand that for the layman the following equations may not make much sense, so after I will explain in plain speech what this means:

In the Planck-Einstein Energy-Frequency Relation, E=hf where E=energy f=frequencies, wavelengths and photon energy and h= what is known as The Planck Constant. Light and energy can be characterized using several spectral quantites, such as frequency v, wavelength λ, wavenumber and their angular equivalents (angular frequency, angular wavelength and angular wavenumber.

These quantities are related through complex equations so that the Planck relation can take a standard form as well as angular forms. The standard forms make use of the Planck constant. The angular forms make use of the reduced Planck constant using the speed of light within the formulas. There is much more details to discuss in this research as well, that cannot fit into this summarized booklet.

WHAT THIS MEANS IN COLLOQUIAL TERMS IS, WE CAN FIND THE ENERGY VALUE OF EVERYTHING IN EXISTENCE, INCLUDING ESSENTIAL OILS AND HUMANS, WITH AN INCREDIBLE ACCURACY, AS WELL AS FIND THEIR ACCURATE POSITIONS ON A SPECTRUM OF QUANTUM LIGHT, KNOWN AS THE ENERGY SPECTRUM.

For an individual, discovering their position on the Energy Spectrum was once considered impossible without help from a physicist, however through the link of quantum studies, we now know that everyone has seen their position on the Energy Spectrum through color upon the spectrum. Until now, researchers did not realize the connection, we know now however, that color has the same numeric values, and can be visualized through prayer or meditation, and the color that an individual can see during these processes is their energy-frequency. Through my method by discovering and mapping energy values of color, Essential Oil energy values, and human energy values, has been the foundation of The Energy Spectrum.

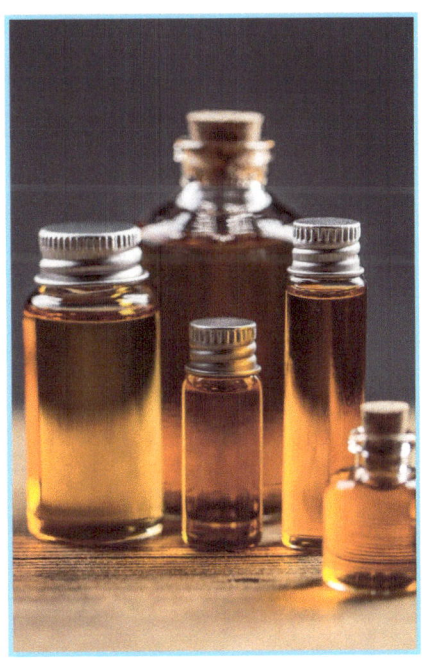

3. IDENTIFYING YOUR POSITION ON THE ENERGY SPECTRUM

In this energy scale, a score between -20 and +20 is considered to be a healthy equilibrium as long as it is counteracted with the same on the opposite side, but it is ideal to achieve 0. 0 signifies a perfect balance within oneself but it is not necessary for all to achieve 0 Balance on their own. Two people, for example, who score -15 and +15 respectively have achieved 0 Balance together, and they are stable and equal within the energies as a team.

Achieving the 0 Balance is an ongoing process, influences can shift you at any and all times. It is important to inspect and evaluate yourself, recognize the effects and causes, and remove the effects of an unwanted weight with a counterweight.

Take notice that within the scale the negative charges are influenced by the light spectrum and 0 Balance is white, or lack of color. These color representations will be important for identifying the essential oils to create the result you desire, and also through your process to identify where you currently lie on the scale. Achieving the 0 Balance can be as simple or as complicated as you desire, you can maintain equilibrium by using a direct counterweight to your position on the Energy Spectrum, or a desired variety of essential oils and load the scale to achieve the balance of 0, on your own or with a partner.

When you pray or meditate, you must put yourself in a place where outer influences are minimized as much as possible so that all the focus can be directed inward to yourself and outward to the spiritual world. It is important to stay within deep focus for at least ten to twenty minutes, and with your eyes closed, what color do you see? What color do you feel? This should tell you where you are on the Energy Spectrum at that moment.

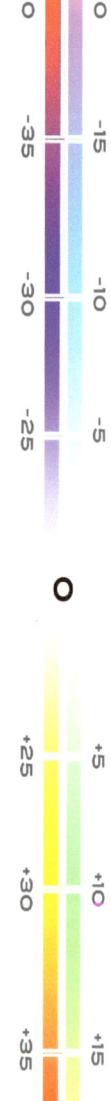

DO YOU SEE A LIGHT BLUE OR A DEEP GREEN? DO YOU FEEL SURROUNDED IN VIOLET?

Does your visualization fluctuate and slide up and down the gradients? Do you see red or black? In the following chapters we will evaluate each color fluctuations and how to counterbalance each one with specific essential oils.

But first, we must categorize the most crucial essential oils along the Energy Spectrum that have been determined as such with their molecular structure and symbiosis within nature and each other.

The D line represents the position of the essential oil if used with diffusion, D = Diffused. A(X) means Application multiplied by X (X = the number of drops used) therefore applying them directly will intensify the affects and more so with the amount that it is directly applied. Think of the Diffused Line as your lighter weights on a standing scale, while the Applied Line are your heavier weights. As you may see, the more drops you use applying the essential oil, the more you are in danger of tipping the Energy Spectrum, or shifting it dramatically. For best results with this method, do not start with the Applied Line, but rather slowly using the Diffused Line counteracting each weight (or energy) with each the other, starting with your own position on the Energy Spectrum, and building a slow and steady harmony between you (or you and a partner) and these natural elements, introducing the Applied line as necessary while always attempting to maintain the 0 Balance.

Each Essential Oil has a specific numeric value that positions itself upon the Energy Spectrum. This numeric value is determined through the chemistry and energetic compounds that each oil possesses. It is true that these essential oils do not have whole number values upon the Energy Spectrum, you'll see that they are rounded to the nearest thousandth to portray them as accurately as possible. There are no essential oils that are completely neutralized, if they were they would possess no effect. However, if you combine all energetic values of the 35 essential oils listed in the this book, their sum is 0 Balance. However, if you add an external element, for example, yourself, into the equation, you affect the equilibrium with your personal Energy Spectrum Position. Please note that a larger energetic value or larger numeric value based on the Energy Spectrum does not imply a stronger aroma. Refer to the appendix to find the exact color position and energetic value

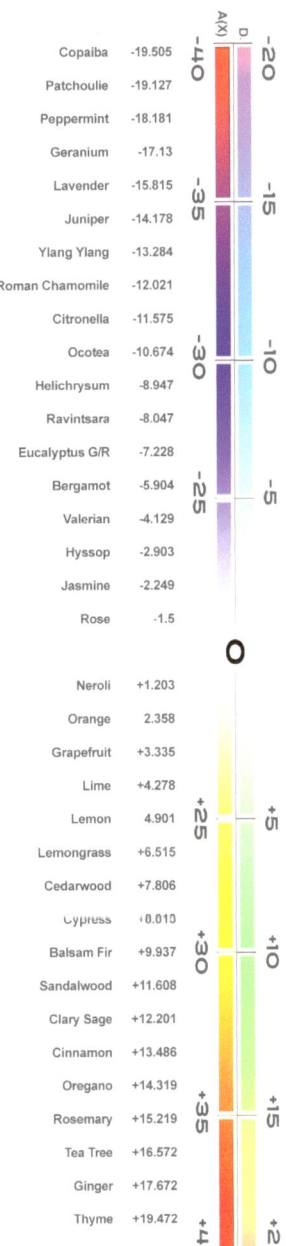

Oil	Value
Copaiba	-19.505
Patchoulie	-19.127
Peppermint	-18.181
Geranium	-17.13
Lavender	-15.815
Juniper	-14.178
Ylang Ylang	-13.284
Roman Chamomile	-12.021
Citronella	-11.575
Ocotea	-10.674
Helichrysum	-8.947
Ravintsara	-8.047
Eucalyptus G/R	-7.228
Bergamot	-5.904
Valerian	-4.129
Hyssop	-2.903
Jasmine	-2.249
Rose	-1.5
Neroli	+1.203
Orange	2.358
Grapefruit	+3.335
Lime	+4.278
Lemon	4.901
Lemongrass	+6.515
Cedarwood	+7.806
Cypress	+8.010
Balsam Fir	+9.937
Sandalwood	+11.608
Clary Sage	+12.201
Cinnamon	+13.486
Oregano	+14.319
Rosemary	+15.219
Tea Tree	+16.572
Ginger	+17.672
Thyme	+19.472
Wintergreen	+20.6

of each essential oil used in this book. Please note that there are other common essential oils that are not referenced in this book, that is because their exact Energy Spectrum positions are still currently under research and study and will be published in the full book version of this summary.

Essential Oils, are created through hydrophobicity, which is the process of gathering the physical property of a molecule. Within water, these molecules attract and cluster together like microscopic magnets. These molecules together form a harmonious aggregate that conglomerate into one composite. The elements within this composite is what it uses to define and charge itself, therefore, whatever molecules are used to create the aggregate, results how the component will affect and directly influence what it is applied to. This is why creating essential oils is a very specific process that has been refined for centuries, one molecule extra or neglected or the wrong combination of molecules can harm the resulting component or set it off balance and thereby affect its usage.

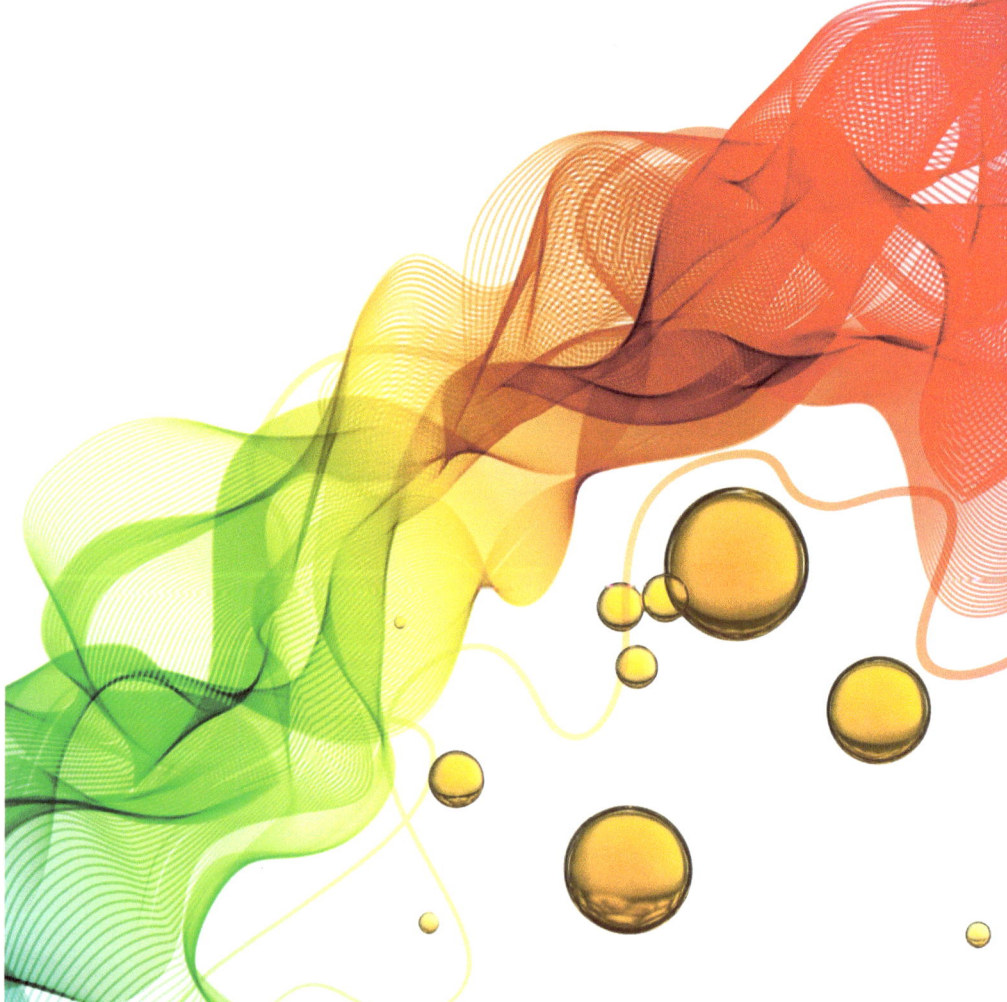

4. ACHIEVING 0 BALANCE

Once you identify your position, you now have a reference point to begin to balance your Energy Spectrum, just as you would use any weight scale, there are a variety of ways to achieve $\underline{0}$ Balance. As you can imagine, there are a million combinations that can be used with this system, it depends on your personal preference and through practice, study and memorization of the color position system, you can become a master at achieving $\underline{0}$ Balance within yourself, with a partner, with multiple partners, or entire crowds in a classroom or therapeutic environment. You can implement this system with your Yoga instruction, prayer meetings, and other gatherings. But first you must master this method with yourself, repeating and refining your methods, referring to the Energy Spectrum as much as possible, until you can achieve $\underline{0}$ Balance relatively easy and responsibly.

COUNTERBALANCING YOUR POSITION WITH ESSENTIAL OILS

To get you started, I wish to give you an example of how this method works. However, for this summary I can only outline two. In the full book version of this sumamry I will go into detail with various positionings as well as practices for counterbalance and methods to introduce The Energy Spectrum into group sessions.

If you visualized very light blue or very light green than you probably feel very calm and at peace, or you are not experiencing extreme emotions at the moment. Things feel right within your world for now and most of your relationships with others and the natural and spiritual worlds are very harmonious. This is of course, your own position within the Energy Spectrum, and you should not attempt to throw the balance off by using an essential oil on the far end of the scale, or being around others who can tip this energy balance, unless of course you counteract it with another essential oil or multiple essential oils that cancel out the added energy. If your partner is experiencing another position on the Energy Spectrum, use graphic2 in the last chapter and pick the essential oils that will create a harmony between you, your partner and the natural and spiritual world.

For a simple balance of a -5 position, diffuse Lemon$^{(+4.9)}$ or a mixture of Neroli$^{(+1.2)}$ and Lime$^{(+4.1)}$, or a mixture of Orange$^{(+2.3)}$ and Grapefruit$^{(+3.1)}$. More complicated mixtures to balance could be used, for example using Lemongrass$^{(+6.4)}$ and Rose$^{(-1.1)}$. Of course, these recipes can be created as complicated as you wish, and more complicated recipes have more precise affects and benefits, but for beginners it is best to start simple.

For a simple balance of +5, diffuse a mix of Valerian$^{(-4.1)}$ and Rose$^{(-1.5)}$.

THIS IS THE FUNDEMENTAL BASICS OF USING THE ENERGY SPECTRUM AND ESSENTIAL OILS TO ACHIEVE 0 BALANCE. USING THE SAME METHOD OF COMBINING ESSENTIAL OIL VALUES, YOU WILL BE ABLE TO BALANCE YOUR ENERGETIC POSITION NO MATTER WHERE IT LANDS UPON THE ENERGY SPECTRUM.

Deep purple or bright orange indicates strong emotions, love, sadness, etc. Not that we cannot feel these emotions while our position is in light blue or medium green, but deep purple or bright orange indicates that these strong emotions are at the forefront of our thoughts at that moment. These emotions are important, and shouldn't be regarded as harmful, we can still feel love while counterbalancing our Energy Spectrum back to $\underline{0}$ balance, or white. When you feel your energy is greater than -25 or +25, this is when the Applied Line of essential oils is better for balance. You have probably felt strong emotions in the past and discovered that when you apply your favorite scent during this time it gives a great feeling of completion. This is all due to the Energy Spectrum. If you are feeling deeply purple, applying a Tea Tree[+16.5] oil behind your ears may compliment your energy. If you see bright orange, Lavender[-15.8] could be used.

5. RED

As I said before, more information and methods of balancing your position will go into greater detail in the full book version of this summary. But, I feel responsibility to inform you of RED positioning.

If you are visualizing Bright Red, then you are very off-balance within the Energy Spectrum. This could be your spiritual or physical body warning you of extreme stress, discomfort or some other disturbance in your life that should be recognized and counterbalanced as soon as possible. But it may also mean deep passion, the tricky part about red is that it is on both ends of the balance of energy making one blind to their position. When you are in the red, it is sometimes difficult to determine whether the disturbance is with positive magnetism or negative magnetism. Diagnosing this correctly is crucial in bringing back balance, and if energy is added on top of the side of your Spectrum that is already lop-sided, it could result in extreme stress and emotional discomfort. But, do not worry, remember the equilibrium of the scale component, for a properly placed energy can give immediate mental comfort. A -40 personal position on the Energy Spectrum will act in perfect harmony with a +40 essential oil counterweight position. The proper method is to slowly add small increments to one side, usually starting with Neroli[+1.2] due to it's lightweight energy, if using Neroli moves your position to purple, you'll know you were too far red on the negative side of the Energy Spectrum and can continue the positive essential oil treatment. If you remain red or become more red while using Neroli, you'll know that you are too far on the positive side, and you can begin counteracting this with Rose[-1.5] and continue the negative essential oil treatment.

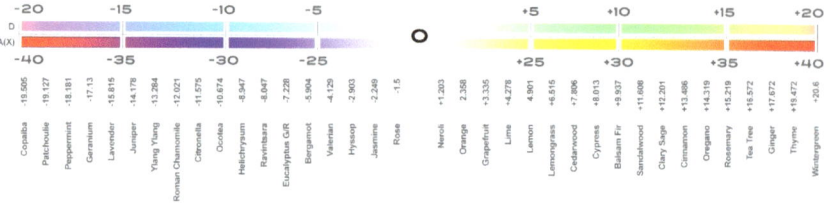

INDEX

This Essential Oil Energy Spectrum Position Values List has been included for your use. Many other Essential Oils have not been included because they are still under research and their energy values have not been discovered to their nearest thousandth decimal as of yet. They will be published in future versions. In summation, these are the numeric values of the energy within essential oils that have been determined through the research methods described in this booklet.

Copaiba	-19.505
Patchoulie	-19.127
Peppermint	-18.181
Geranium	-17.13
Lavender	-15.815
Juniper	-14.178
Ylang Ylang	-13.284
Roman Chamomile	-12.021
Citronella	-11.575
Ocotea	-10.674
Helichrysum	-8.947
Ravintsara	-8.047
Eucalyptus G/R	-7.228
Bergamot	-5.904
Valerian	-4.129
Hyssop	-2.903
Jasmine	-2.249
Rose	-1.5
Neroli	+1.203
Orange	+2.358
Grapefruit	+3.335
Lime	+4.278
Lemon	+4.901
Lemongrass	+6.515
Cedarwood	+7.806
Cypress	+8.013
Balsam Fir	+9.937
Sandalwood	+11.608
Clary Sage	+12.201
Cinnamon	+13.486
Oregano	+14.319
Rosemary	+15.219
Tea Tree	+16.572
Ginger	+17.672
Thyme	+19.472
Wintergreen	+20.6

-40 -20
-35 -15
-30 -10
-25 -5

0

+25 +5
+30 +10
+35 +15
+40 +20

PROGRESS NOTES

PROGRESS NOTES

PROGRESS NOTES

PROGRESS NOTES

PROGRESS NOTES

PROGRESS NOTES

PROGRESS NOTES

PROGRESS NOTES

PROGRESS NOTES

PROGRESS NOTES

PROGRESS NOTES

PROGRESS NOTES

PROGRESS NOTES

PROGRESS NOTES

www.ingramcontent.com/pod-product-compliance
Lightning Source LLC
Chambersburg PA
CBHW050933290526
45792CB00002B/995